The Sound Guardian: Safeguarding Your Hearing in a Noisy World

David Henry

Copyright © [2023]

Title: The Sound Guardian: Safeguarding Your Hearing in a Noisy World
Author's: David Henry

All rights reserved. No part of this publication may be reproduced, stored in a retrieval system, or transmitted in any form or by any means, electronic, mechanical, photocopying, recording, or otherwise, without the prior written permission of the publisher or author, except in the case of brief quotations embodied in critical reviews and certain other non-commercial uses permitted by copyright law.

This book was printed and published by [Publisher's: **David Henry**] in [2023]

ISBN:

TABLE OF CONTENT

Chapter 1: Introduction to Hearing Conservation   07

The Importance of Protecting Your Hearing

Understanding How Hearing Works

Common Causes of Hearing Loss

The Impact of Noise on Hearing Health

Chapter 2: The Basics of Noise-Induced Hearing Loss   16

What is Noise-Induced Hearing Loss?

How Noise-Induced Hearing Loss Occurs

Signs and Symptoms of Noise-Induced Hearing Loss

Identifying High-Risk Environments

Chapter 3: Understanding Ear Anatomy   24

The Structure and Function of the Ear

The Role of Each Ear Component in Hearing

Common Ear Conditions and Disorders

Chapter 4: Assessing Noise Levels   30

Measuring Noise Levels

Understanding Decibel (dB) Ratings

Recognizing Safe and Unsafe Noise Levels

Noise Assessment Tools and Devices

Chapter 5: Types of Hearing Protection   38

Earplugs: Pros and Cons

Earmuffs: Pros and Cons

Custom-Made Ear Protection

Choosing the Right Hearing Protection for Different Situations

Chapter 6: Proper Usage and Maintenance of Hearing Protection   46

How to Wear Earplugs Correctly

Putting on and Adjusting Earmuffs

Cleaning and Maintaining Hearing Protection Devices

Ensuring a Proper Fit for Custom-Made Ear Protection

Chapter 7: Strategies for Hearing Conservation   54

Creating a Hearing Conservation Program

Implementing Engineering Controls to Reduce Noise

Administrative Controls for Hearing Protection

Personal Protective Equipment (PPE) Policies and Procedures

Chapter 8: The Role of Education and Awareness   63

Spreading Awareness about Hearing Conservation

Educating Employees, Students, and the General Public

Promoting Hearing Health in the Community

The Importance of Regular Hearing Check-ups

Chapter 9: The Future of Ear Protection 71

Advancements in Hearing Protection Technology

Potential Innovations in Noise Reduction

Research and Development in Hearing Conservation

Promising Strategies for Future Ear Protection

Chapter 10: Conclusion and Resources 80

Recap of Key Points

Additional Resources for Hearing Conservation

Taking Action: Steps Towards Protecting Your Hearing

Final Thoughts and Encouragement for Safeguarding Your Hearing

Chapter 1: Introduction to Hearing Conservation

The Importance of Protecting Your Hearing

Introduction:
Welcome to "The Sound Guardian: Safeguarding Your Hearing in a Noisy World." In this subchapter, we will explore the significance of protecting your hearing and the impact it can have on your overall well-being. Whether you are a music lover, a sports enthusiast, or simply someone who cherishes the sounds of nature, understanding the importance of preserving your ears becomes vital. So, let's dive into the world of healthy hearing!

The Marvels of the Ears:
Our ears are extraordinary organs that enable us to perceive the world around us. They allow us to enjoy the beauty of music, engage in conversations, and even detect potential dangers. However, we often take them for granted, exposing them to loud noises without realizing the long-term consequences.

The Risks of Noise Exposure:
Did you know that prolonged exposure to loud noises can cause irreversible damage to our hearing? This damage, known as noise-induced hearing loss, can lead to difficulties in communication, social isolation, and even mental health issues. It is essential to be aware of the risks associated with excessive noise and take measures to protect our ears from harm.

Prevention is the Key:
Protecting your hearing is a lifelong commitment that begins with

simple yet effective precautions. The first step is education – understanding the decibel levels of common noises and identifying potential sources of excessive noise in your daily life. By being aware, you can take proactive measures such as using earplugs or earmuffs to reduce noise exposure.

Promoting Healthy Habits:
In addition to taking precautions, adopting healthy habits can significantly contribute to maintaining good hearing. Regular breaks from noisy environments, limiting the use of headphones or earbuds, and keeping the volume at a safe level are all essential practices. Furthermore, incorporating a balanced diet and exercise routine can improve blood circulation to the ears, enhancing their overall health.

The Role of Technology:
In today's world, technology plays a significant role in our lives. However, it is crucial to be mindful of its potential impact on our hearing. Listening to music at high volumes through headphones or attending loud concerts can damage our ears. Utilizing noise-canceling headphones and following recommended volume levels can help protect your ears while still enjoying the benefits of modern technology.

Conclusion:
Protecting your hearing is a responsibility that benefits everyone, regardless of age or occupation. By understanding the risks associated with noise exposure, taking preventive measures, and adopting healthy habits, we can ensure the longevity of our precious ears. Remember, healthy hearing is not only a gift but also a gateway to experiencing the

world in all its captivating sounds. So, let us embark on this journey together and become guardians of our hearing!

Understanding How Hearing Works

Our sense of hearing is truly remarkable, allowing us to perceive and interpret a rich tapestry of sounds that surround us. Whether it's the melodic notes of a song, the gentle rustling of leaves, or the laughter of loved ones, our ears play a crucial role in our daily lives. In this subchapter, we will delve into the fascinating world of auditory perception and explore the inner workings of our ears.

The ear is a complex and intricate organ, consisting of three main parts: the outer ear, the middle ear, and the inner ear. Each component plays a unique role in the process of hearing, working together seamlessly to deliver sound signals to our brain.

The journey of sound begins in the outer ear, where sound waves are collected and channeled towards the eardrum. As sound waves enter the ear canal, they vibrate the eardrum, which in turn sets off a chain reaction in the middle ear.

In the middle ear, three tiny bones called ossicles, namely the malleus, incus, and stapes, amplify and transmit the vibrations from the eardrum to the inner ear. This amplification process is essential for maintaining the clarity and fidelity of the sound.

Once the vibrations reach the inner ear, they encounter a fluid-filled structure called the cochlea. The cochlea is lined with thousands of tiny hair cells that transform the mechanical vibrations into electrical signals, which can be interpreted by our brain as sound.

These electrical signals travel through the auditory nerve to the brain, where they are decoded and transformed into meaningful sounds. The brain processes and interprets these signals, allowing us to identify and differentiate various sounds, such as speech, music, and environmental noises.

Understanding how hearing works is crucial for safeguarding our auditory health. By appreciating the delicate mechanisms of our ears, we can take proactive steps to protect them from potential hazards. From using hearing protection in noisy environments to seeking timely medical attention for any signs of hearing loss, we can ensure the longevity of our hearing abilities.

In conclusion, our ears are incredible organs that enable us to experience the world of sound. By understanding the intricate process of hearing, we can appreciate the importance of preserving our auditory health. So, let us embark on this journey together, as we explore the wonders of hearing and learn how to be sound guardians of our ears in this noisy world.

Common Causes of Hearing Loss

Hearing loss is a common problem that affects people of all ages and can significantly impact their quality of life. Understanding the causes of hearing loss is essential for everyone, as it empowers individuals to take necessary steps to safeguard their hearing in a noisy world. In this subchapter, we will explore some of the most common causes of hearing loss and provide valuable insights to help preserve the health of our ears.

One of the leading causes of hearing loss is prolonged exposure to loud noise. Whether it's from attending concerts, using headphones at high volumes, or working in noisy environments, the delicate structures in our ears can become damaged over time. This type of hearing loss, known as noise-induced hearing loss, is preventable by practicing safe listening habits, such as using hearing protection devices and taking regular breaks from loud environments.

Age-related hearing loss, also known as presbycusis, is another prevalent cause of hearing loss. As we age, the sensory cells in our inner ears gradually deteriorate, leading to a gradual decline in hearing ability. While age-related hearing loss is a natural part of the aging process, there are lifestyle factors that can accelerate its progression. By adopting a healthy lifestyle, avoiding excessive noise exposure, and managing underlying health conditions, we can minimize the impact of age-related hearing loss.

Certain medical conditions and medications can also contribute to hearing loss. Conditions like otosclerosis, which affects the movement of the tiny bones in the middle ear, and Ménière's disease, a disorder of the inner ear, can lead to varying degrees of hearing loss. Additionally, certain medications, including some antibiotics and chemotherapy drugs, have the potential to damage the auditory system. It is crucial to be aware of the potential side effects of medications and consult with healthcare professionals when necessary.

Lastly, ear infections, particularly in children, can cause temporary or permanent hearing loss if left untreated. Middle ear infections can lead to fluid buildup, which interferes with sound transmission and affects hearing. Prompt diagnosis and appropriate treatment of ear infections are vital in preventing long-term hearing loss.

By understanding the common causes of hearing loss, we can make informed decisions to protect our ears and preserve our hearing. Whether it's adopting safe listening practices, managing health conditions, or seeking timely medical attention, taking proactive measures is crucial in safeguarding our hearing in a noisy world. Remember, our hearing health is a precious gift that deserves our attention and care.

The Impact of Noise on Hearing Health

Noise is an inevitable part of our daily lives, whether it's the bustling city streets, blaring music at concerts, or even the hum of appliances in our homes. While we may not always pay attention to the impact noise can have on our hearing health, it is crucial to understand and protect our ears from potential damage.

Exposure to excessive noise can lead to various hearing problems, such as temporary or permanent hearing loss, tinnitus (a persistent ringing or buzzing in the ears), and hyperacusis (an increased sensitivity to sound). These conditions can significantly impact our quality of life, making it difficult to communicate, enjoy music, or even sleep peacefully.

One of the primary reasons noise poses a threat to our hearing health is the decibel level. Sounds above 85 decibels (dB) can cause damage to the delicate structures of our ears. To put it into perspective, a typical conversation measures around 60 dB, while the sound of a rock concert can exceed 100 dB. Prolonged exposure to high decibel levels can gradually erode the cells responsible for our hearing, leading to irreversible damage.

It is not just the intensity of noise that affects our ears but also the duration of exposure. A brief exposure to a loud sound may not cause immediate harm, but repeated exposure or prolonged exposure to moderate noise levels can accumulate damage over time. This is why it is essential to be aware of the noise levels in our environment and take necessary precautions to protect our hearing.

Fortunately, there are several steps we can take to safeguard our hearing in this noisy world. One of the simplest and most effective ways is to use ear protection, such as earplugs or earmuffs, in high-noise environments. This can significantly reduce the decibel levels reaching our ears and prevent potential damage.

Additionally, we should strive to limit our exposure to loud noises whenever possible. This can be achieved by keeping the volume at a reasonable level while listening to music or watching television, taking breaks in quiet areas during events or parties, and avoiding noisy activities for extended periods.

Regular hearing check-ups are another crucial aspect of maintaining hearing health. By monitoring our hearing abilities, we can detect any changes early on and take appropriate action to prevent further damage.

In conclusion, noise has a profound impact on our hearing health. Understanding the potential risks and taking proactive measures to protect our ears is essential for everyone. By wearing ear protection, limiting exposure to loud noises, and getting regular check-ups, we can safeguard our hearing and enjoy a world filled with beautiful sounds without compromising our long-term auditory well-being.

Chapter 2: The Basics of Noise-Induced Hearing Loss

What is Noise-Induced Hearing Loss?

In the bustling world we live in, our ears are constantly bombarded with a symphony of sounds. From the noise of traffic to the blaring music at concerts, our ears are exposed to a range of decibels that can have lasting effects on our hearing. This subchapter aims to shed light on the concept of noise-induced hearing loss and the importance of safeguarding our ears in a noisy world.

Noise-induced hearing loss refers to a type of hearing impairment caused by prolonged exposure to loud sounds. Unlike other forms of hearing loss, which may be caused by genetic factors or aging, noise-induced hearing loss is entirely preventable. It occurs when the delicate hair cells in our inner ear are damaged or destroyed due to excessive noise levels.

The human ear is a remarkable organ. It can perceive a wide range of sounds, from the softest whispers to the loudest explosions. However, when exposed to sounds above 85 decibels for an extended period, our ears become vulnerable to damage. This is roughly equivalent to the noise produced by heavy traffic, construction sites, or even a rock concert.

The symptoms of noise-induced hearing loss may not be immediately apparent. Initially, one may experience a temporary loss of hearing or a sensation of muffled sounds after exposure to loud noises. However, if these warning signs are consistently ignored, the damage becomes irreversible, resulting in permanent hearing loss.

Protecting our ears is crucial, and there are practical steps we can take to safeguard our hearing. Investing in high-quality ear protection, such as earplugs or earmuffs, can significantly reduce the risk of noise-induced hearing loss. Limiting exposure to loud noises, taking breaks in quiet environments, and keeping the volume at a moderate level when using headphones are also essential precautions to take.

In conclusion, noise-induced hearing loss is a preventable form of hearing impairment caused by prolonged exposure to loud sounds. By understanding the risks associated with excessive noise levels and taking proactive measures to protect our ears, we can ensure our hearing remains intact. Let us be sound guardians in this noisy world, preserving our hearing and enjoying the melodies of life for years to come.

How Noise-Induced Hearing Loss Occurs

In today's bustling world, our ears are constantly bombarded with various sounds and noises. From the blaring horns of traffic to the loud music at concerts, our ears are constantly under siege. However, few of us stop to consider the potential consequences of this daily assault on our hearing. Noise-induced hearing loss (NIHL) is an alarming condition that affects millions of people worldwide. In this subchapter, we will delve into how NIHL occurs and the steps we can take to safeguard our precious hearing.

NIHL occurs when our ears are exposed to excessive noise levels, causing damage to the delicate structures within the ear. The loudness of a sound is measured in units called decibels (dB). Prolonged exposure to sounds above 85 dB can lead to irreversible hearing damage. Concerts, construction sites, and even everyday activities like using power tools or listening to music through headphones at high volumes can all contribute to NIHL.

The inner ear is composed of tiny hair cells that are responsible for transmitting sound signals to the brain. When exposed to loud noises, these hair cells become damaged or destroyed. Initially, the damage may be temporary, resulting in a temporary threshold shift (TTS), where hearing returns to normal after a period of rest. However, repeated exposure to loud noises can cause permanent damage, resulting in a permanent threshold shift (PTS). PTS leads to a gradual loss of hearing over time, often starting with high-frequency sounds.

Preventing NIHL is crucial for maintaining good hearing health. One of the most effective ways to prevent NIHL is to reduce exposure to loud noises. This can be achieved by wearing ear protection, such as earmuffs or earplugs, in noisy environments. It is also essential to give your ears regular breaks from loud noises and to keep the volume at a safe level when using headphones or attending concerts.

Educating ourselves and others about the dangers of excessive noise exposure is equally important. By spreading awareness, we can encourage individuals to take proactive steps to protect their hearing. Additionally, regular hearing screenings can help identify any signs of hearing loss and allow for early intervention.

In conclusion, noise-induced hearing loss is a prevalent and preventable condition that affects individuals of all ages. By understanding how NIHL occurs and implementing preventative measures, we can safeguard our hearing in this noisy world. Remember, your ears are precious and deserve to be protected.

Signs and Symptoms of Noise-Induced Hearing Loss

Noise-induced hearing loss is a common yet preventable condition that affects people of all ages. In this subchapter, we will explore the signs and symptoms of this type of hearing loss, which can help you identify if you or someone you know is at risk.

One of the most noticeable signs of noise-induced hearing loss is difficulty in understanding speech, especially in noisy environments. You may find yourself struggling to follow conversations or constantly asking others to repeat themselves. This can lead to frustration and social isolation if left untreated.

Another key symptom is a persistent ringing, buzzing, or roaring sound in the ears, known as tinnitus. Tinnitus can vary in intensity and may be continuous or occasional. If you experience this symptom, it is essential to seek medical attention as it can significantly impact your quality of life.

Gradual hearing loss over time is also a common symptom of noise-induced hearing loss. You may notice that certain sounds, such as birds chirping or the doorbell ringing, become increasingly difficult to hear. This type of hearing loss typically affects high-frequency sounds first, making it harder to detect.

In some cases, noise-induced hearing loss can be accompanied by feelings of fullness or pressure in the ears. This sensation, known as ear blockage, can occur due to damage to the delicate structures within the ear caused by exposure to loud noise. If you frequently experience this symptom, it is essential to consult with an audiologist for a comprehensive hearing evaluation.

It is important to note that the signs and symptoms of noise-induced hearing loss can vary from person to person. Some individuals may experience only mild symptoms, while others may have more severe hearing loss. Regardless of the severity, seeking early intervention and treatment is crucial to prevent further damage and improve your overall hearing health.

In conclusion, understanding the signs and symptoms of noise-induced hearing loss is essential for everyone, regardless of age or niche. By being aware of these indicators, you can take necessary steps to protect your ears from excessive noise exposure and seek appropriate medical attention if you suspect hearing loss. Remember, safeguarding your hearing is a lifelong commitment, and early intervention is key to preserving your auditory well-being.

Identifying High-Risk Environments

Introduction:
In our modern, bustling world, our ears are constantly exposed to a barrage of noise. From bustling city streets to busy workplaces, it is essential to identify high-risk environments that can potentially damage our hearing. In this subchapter, we will discuss the importance of recognizing these environments and provide you with valuable tips on how to protect your ears in such settings. Whether you are a student, professional, or simply someone who cares about their hearing, understanding the risks and taking preventive measures is crucial for maintaining healthy ears.

Understanding High-Risk Environments:
High-risk environments refer to places where noise levels exceed safe limits and can pose a threat to our hearing health. These environments can include construction sites, live music venues, airports, and even some recreational activities like shooting ranges or motorsports events. It is imperative to recognize these settings to avoid long-term damage to our ears.

Recognizing the Warning Signs:
Identifying high-risk environments is not always straightforward. However, there are some tell-tale signs that can help you determine if you are in a potentially hazardous soundscape. These signs include having to raise your voice to be heard, feeling discomfort or pain in your ears, or experiencing temporary hearing loss or ringing in your ears after leaving the environment. Being aware of these indicators will enable you to take immediate action to protect your ears.

Protecting Your Ears:
To safeguard your hearing in high-risk environments, it is essential to take proactive measures. One of the most effective solutions is wearing hearing protection devices, such as earplugs or earmuffs. These devices can significantly reduce the intensity of sound and protect your ears from potential damage. Additionally, maintaining a safe distance from loud sources and taking regular breaks in quieter areas can help minimize the risk of long-term hearing loss.

Education and Advocacy:
As an advocate for ear health, it is crucial to educate others about the risks associated with high-noise environments. By spreading awareness and encouraging others to take necessary precautions, we can create a safer and more hearing-conscious society. Remember, protecting your ears is a responsibility we all share.

Conclusion:
Identifying high-risk environments and understanding the potential dangers they pose to our hearing is vital for maintaining healthy ears. By recognizing warning signs, taking preventive measures, and advocating for ear health, we can protect our hearing and ensure a better quality of life. Together, let us become sound guardians in this noisy world, safeguarding our precious gift of hearing for ourselves and future generations.

Chapter 3: Understanding Ear Anatomy

The Structure and Function of the Ear

Understanding the intricate structure and function of the ear is essential for safeguarding our hearing in today's noisy world. The ear is not just a simple organ responsible for hearing; it is a complex system that plays a vital role in our overall well-being. In this subchapter, we will explore the various components of the ear and their functions, offering valuable insights for everyone concerned about their auditory health.

The ear can be divided into three main parts: the outer ear, middle ear, and inner ear. Each section has unique structures and functions that contribute to our ability to hear and maintain balance.

Starting with the outer ear, which is the visible part of our ear, it consists of the pinna and the ear canal. The pinna helps collect sound waves and directs them into the ear canal. The ear canal, in turn, channels the sound waves to the eardrum, a thin membrane that separates the outer and middle ear.

Moving on to the middle ear, we encounter the three smallest bones in the human body: the malleus, incus, and stapes, collectively known as the ossicles. These bones transmit sound vibrations from the eardrum to the inner ear. Additionally, the middle ear houses the Eustachian tube, responsible for equalizing pressure between the middle ear and the outside environment.

Finally, we arrive at the inner ear, a complex structure that contains the cochlea, vestibule, and semicircular canals. The cochlea is responsible for converting sound vibrations into electrical signals that can be interpreted by the brain. The vestibule and semicircular canals play a crucial role in maintaining balance and spatial orientation.

Understanding the structure of the ear is only part of the equation. We must also comprehend how each component functions to appreciate the delicate nature of our hearing. By gaining insights into the function of the outer, middle, and inner ear, we can take proactive steps to protect our hearing from the damaging effects of excessive noise exposure.

In conclusion, the structure and function of the ear are crucial elements to consider when it comes to safeguarding our hearing. Being aware of the intricate mechanisms that allow us to hear and maintain balance empowers us to make informed decisions to protect our precious auditory health. Whether you are an audiophile, musician, or simply someone who values their hearing, understanding the ear's structure and function is essential in today's noisy world.

The Role of Each Ear Component in Hearing

Understanding the intricate workings of the ear is essential to safeguarding your hearing in a noisy world. Our ears are remarkably complex organs that enable us to experience the rich tapestry of sounds that surround us. In this subchapter, we will delve into the role of each ear component in the process of hearing.

The outer ear, consisting of the pinna and the ear canal, plays a crucial role in capturing sound waves. The pinna, the visible part of the ear, acts as a funnel, collecting sound and directing it into the ear canal. The ear canal, a narrow passage leading to the middle ear, amplifies and filters the sound waves before they reach the eardrum.

Moving deeper into the ear, we encounter the middle ear, which contains the ossicles. These three tiny bones, namely the malleus, incus, and stapes, are responsible for transmitting sound vibrations from the eardrum to the inner ear. The malleus is attached to the eardrum and transfers its vibrations to the incus, which, in turn, passes them to the stapes. The stapes then transmits the vibrations to the inner ear through a small opening called the oval window.

Within the inner ear lies the cochlea, a spiral-shaped organ filled with fluid and lined with tiny hair cells. These hair cells play a critical role in converting sound vibrations into electrical signals that can be interpreted by the brain. As sound waves pass through the fluid-filled cochlea, they cause the hair cells to bend. This bending triggers the release of neurotransmitters, initiating the transmission of electrical signals to the auditory nerve.

The auditory nerve carries these electrical signals to the brain, specifically to the auditory cortex, where they are decoded into meaningful sounds. This remarkable process allows us to appreciate the nuances of music, comprehend speech, and remain attuned to our surroundings.

Understanding the role of each ear component empowers us to protect our hearing. By recognizing the vulnerability of our ears to excessive noise, we can take proactive measures to minimize exposure and prevent hearing loss. From using ear protection in loud environments to practicing safe listening habits, we can safeguard our hearing and preserve this precious sense for years to come.

In conclusion, our ears are marvels of engineering, with each component playing a vital role in the process of hearing. By appreciating the functions of the outer ear, middle ear, inner ear, and auditory nerve, we can better understand the importance of protecting our hearing and maintaining a healthy auditory system.

Common Ear Conditions and Disorders

Our ears are remarkable organs that allow us to experience the beauty of sound. However, like any other part of our body, they are susceptible to various conditions and disorders. In this subchapter, we will explore some of the most common ear conditions and disorders, aiming to increase awareness and understanding among everyone, regardless of age or background.

One prevalent condition is earwax buildup, also known as cerumen impaction. Earwax is a natural substance that helps protect our ears by trapping dust and debris. However, excessive wax can accumulate and lead to discomfort, hearing loss, or even ear infections. We will discuss preventive measures and safe methods to remove excess earwax, ensuring optimal ear health.

Another common issue affecting our ears is otitis media, commonly known as an ear infection. This condition often occurs in children, but it can also affect adults. We will delve into the causes, symptoms, and treatment options for ear infections, emphasizing the importance of early detection and proper medical care.

Tinnitus, a condition characterized by persistent ringing or buzzing sounds in the ears, affects millions of people worldwide. We will shed light on the potential causes of tinnitus, including exposure to loud noises, age-related hearing loss, and certain medical conditions. Moreover, we will explore both medical and lifestyle-based management techniques to help alleviate the symptoms and improve quality of life for those experiencing tinnitus.

Additionally, we cannot overlook the impact of noise-induced hearing loss, a common disorder that results from prolonged exposure to excessive noise levels. We will discuss the various sources of noise pollution in our daily lives and offer practical tips on how to protect our ears from irreversible damage. By raising awareness about the importance of ear protection and providing guidance, we aim to empower individuals to make informed decisions regarding their hearing health.

Finally, we will touch upon other lesser-known ear conditions, such as Meniere's disease, which causes episodes of vertigo, hearing loss, and tinnitus. By providing an overview of these conditions and their symptoms, we hope to encourage individuals to seek professional help and support when needed.

In conclusion, this subchapter serves as a comprehensive guide to common ear conditions and disorders. By enhancing our knowledge about these issues, we can take proactive measures to safeguard our hearing and maintain optimal ear health. Whether you are a parent concerned about your child's ear health or an adult experiencing hearing-related challenges, this information will prove invaluable in navigating the intricacies of ear conditions and disorders. Remember, protecting our ears is not only crucial for our present well-being but also for our future quality of life.

Chapter 4: Assessing Noise Levels

Measuring Noise Levels

In our modern, bustling world, noise has become an inescapable part of our daily lives. Whether it's the honking of cars, the hum of machinery, or the blaring music in our headphones, we are constantly surrounded by a cacophony of sounds. However, what many of us fail to realize is the potential harm that excessive noise can have on our precious ears. This subchapter, "Measuring Noise Levels," aims to provide you with the knowledge and tools necessary to safeguard your hearing in this noisy world.

Understanding the intensity of sound is crucial in gauging its potential harm. Sound is measured in units called decibels (dB). The higher the decibel level, the louder the sound. Prolonged exposure to sounds above 85 dB can cause irreversible damage to your ears, leading to hearing loss. Therefore, it is essential to be able to measure noise levels accurately.

One of the most common tools for measuring noise levels is a sound level meter. This device detects and quantifies sound pressure levels in decibels. With a sound level meter, you can assess the noise levels in your environment and take appropriate measures to protect your ears. These meters are available in various models, ranging from simple handheld devices to more sophisticated ones used by professionals.

When measuring noise levels, it is crucial to consider the duration of exposure. The Occupational Safety and Health Administration (OSHA) has set guidelines to protect workers from excessive noise exposure. According to these guidelines, exposure to noise levels above 85 dB for more than eight hours can be hazardous. For every increase of 3 dB, the permissible exposure time is reduced by half. So, if the noise level reaches 88 dB, the recommended exposure time decreases to four hours. By understanding these guidelines, you can make informed decisions about how long you expose yourself to different noise levels.

Additionally, there are smartphone apps available that can measure sound levels. These apps utilize your phone's microphone to detect and analyze the noise around you. While they may not be as accurate as professional sound level meters, they can still provide a good estimate of the noise levels in your immediate surroundings.

By measuring noise levels, you gain the power to make informed decisions about protecting your ears. Whether it's using earplugs or noise-canceling headphones, adjusting the volume on your devices, or taking regular breaks from loud environments, being aware of the noise levels can help you safeguard your hearing in this noisy world.

Remember, your ears are precious and deserve to be protected. Take control of your sound environment, measure the noise levels, and take the necessary steps to preserve your hearing for a lifetime of sound enjoyment.

Understanding Decibel (dB) Ratings

When it comes to protecting our ears, understanding decibel (dB) ratings is essential. The decibel scale measures sound intensity and allows us to quantify the potential harm that loud sounds can inflict on our delicate ears. In this subchapter, we will dive into the world of decibels and explore how they affect our hearing.

To put it simply, decibels are units used to measure the volume or intensity of sound. The scale is logarithmic, meaning that each increase of 10 dB represents a tenfold increase in sound intensity. For example, a sound measuring 60 dB is ten times louder than one measuring 50 dB. This logarithmic nature highlights just how sensitive our ears are to even slight changes in sound levels.

Understanding decibel ratings is particularly important for everyone, as our ears are constantly exposed to various noise sources in our everyday lives. From traffic noise to loud music at concerts, our ears can be subject to damaging levels of sound if we are not careful. Prolonged exposure to sounds above 85 dB can lead to noise-induced hearing loss, a condition that is both preventable and irreversible.

To put things into perspective, a whisper is around 30 dB, while a normal conversation clocks in at approximately 60 dB. On the other end of the scale, a jet engine taking off can reach a staggering 140 dB. It is crucial to understand that any sound above 85 dB has the potential to cause damage, especially if exposure is prolonged or repeated.

Knowing the decibel ratings of common noise sources can help us make informed decisions to protect our ears. Whether it's wearing earplugs at a concert or using noise-cancelling headphones in a noisy environment, taking proactive steps can prevent long-term damage to our hearing.

Additionally, it is important to note that decibel ratings are not solely about volume. Different frequencies can affect our ears differently. For example, high-frequency sounds like a screeching whistle can be more damaging than low-frequency sounds such as a bass-heavy music track. This is why understanding decibel ratings in relation to frequency is crucial in safeguarding our hearing.

In conclusion, understanding decibel ratings is vital for everyone to protect our ears from potential harm. By being aware of the intensity of different sounds and their potential impact on our hearing, we can make informed choices to safeguard our ears in a noisy world. Remember, prevention is always better than cure when it comes to our hearing health.

Recognizing Safe and Unsafe Noise Levels

Protecting our hearing is crucial in today's noisy world. With the constant barrage of sounds from traffic, construction, and electronic devices, it's imperative to understand the difference between safe and unsafe noise levels. This subchapter aims to help everyone, regardless of age or background, recognize and navigate the vast range of sound exposures that can impact our ears.

Firstly, it's essential to understand the concept of decibels (dB), the unit used to measure sound intensity. A whisper typically registers at around 30 dB, while a jet engine can reach a staggering 140 dB. Experts agree that prolonged exposure to sounds above 85 dB can cause irreversible damage to our ears, leading to hearing loss or tinnitus. By recognizing the safe and unsafe noise thresholds, we can take proactive measures to safeguard our hearing.

Recognizing safe noise levels is the first step towards hearing preservation. Everyday sounds like conversations, television volume, and normal office noises are usually within the safe range of 60-70 dB. However, it's crucial to remember that even continuous exposure to sounds at this level can gradually impact our hearing. By being aware of the volume levels around us, we can make conscious decisions to reduce excessive noise, such as lowering the volume on our headphones or using earplugs in loud environments.

On the other hand, recognizing unsafe noise levels is equally important to protect our ears from harm. Activities that generate loud sounds, such as attending concerts, using power tools, or riding motorcycles, often exceed the safe threshold. It's vital to take precautions, such as wearing ear protection devices like earmuffs or earplugs, to minimize the risk of damage. Additionally, maintaining a safe distance from sources of loud noise can significantly reduce our exposure.

Children, in particular, need extra attention when it comes to recognizing safe and unsafe noise levels. Their developing ears are more susceptible to damage, and it's our responsibility to monitor their sound environment. Parents, teachers, and caregivers should educate themselves about safe noise levels for children and ensure that they are not exposed to loud noises for extended periods.

By recognizing safe and unsafe noise levels, we can proactively protect our ears and preserve our hearing for years to come. It is essential for everyone to be aware of the potential risks associated with excessive noise exposure and to take appropriate measures to minimize these risks. Remember, your ears are invaluable, and their protection is in your hands.

Noise Assessment Tools and Devices

In today's fast-paced world, we are constantly exposed to various sources of noise that can potentially harm our hearing. Whether it's the blaring horns of traffic, the booming music at concerts, or the constant chatter in a crowded restaurant, our ears are under constant assault. As a result, it is crucial for everyone to be aware of the potential risks and take steps to protect their hearing. This subchapter focuses on noise assessment tools and devices that can help us measure and monitor the noise levels in our environment.

One of the most common tools for noise assessment is a sound level meter. This handheld device measures the intensity of sound waves in decibels (dB). Sound level meters are easy to use and provide accurate readings, allowing individuals to determine if the noise levels around them are safe or potentially damaging. With the help of these devices, we can make informed decisions about our exposure to different environments and take appropriate measures to protect our hearing.

Another useful device is a personal noise dosimeter. These small, portable devices are worn by individuals to measure their personal exposure to noise over a specific period. Noise dosimeters provide valuable information about the cumulative noise levels experienced by an individual, taking into account both the intensity and duration of exposure. By using these devices, individuals can gain a better understanding of their overall noise exposure and make necessary adjustments in their daily routines to minimize the risk of hearing damage.

For those who work in noisy environments, such as construction sites or factories, the use of noise monitoring systems is essential. These systems consist of multiple noise sensors strategically placed throughout the workplace, continuously measuring and recording the noise levels. By analyzing the data collected, employers can identify areas with excessive noise and take appropriate measures to mitigate the risks. This ensures a safer working environment for employees and reduces the chances of occupational hearing loss.

In addition to these tools, there are also smartphone applications available that can serve as noise assessment tools. These apps use the built-in microphone of the device to measure noise levels and provide real-time feedback. While not as accurate as professional devices, they can still be useful for individuals to get a general idea of the noise levels in their surroundings.

By utilizing noise assessment tools and devices, we can take proactive steps to safeguard our hearing. These tools provide us with the information we need to make informed decisions about our exposure to noise, allowing us to protect our ears and prevent hearing loss. Remember, our hearing is precious, and it is our responsibility to take care of it in this noisy world.

Chapter 5: Types of Hearing Protection

Earplugs: Pros and Cons

In today's modern and bustling world, our ears are constantly bombarded with all sorts of noises. From the blaring horns of traffic to the loud music in clubs and concerts, our delicate sense of hearing is under constant assault. This is why it is crucial to take proactive steps to protect our ears, and one effective solution is the use of earplugs. In this subchapter, we will explore the pros and cons of using earplugs to safeguard your hearing in a noisy world.

On the positive side, earplugs offer a range of benefits. Firstly, they provide a physical barrier that reduces the intensity of sound reaching your eardrums. By blocking out excessive noise, earplugs help prevent temporary or permanent hearing damage, allowing you to enjoy activities without compromising your auditory health. Additionally, earplugs are portable, convenient, and readily available in various sizes and materials, making them a practical solution for anyone seeking to protect their ears.

Furthermore, earplugs can be especially advantageous for individuals who work or live in loud environments. Construction workers, musicians, and frequent concert-goers can greatly benefit from wearing earplugs regularly. By reducing noise exposure, earplugs can prevent noise-induced hearing loss, tinnitus, and other auditory problems that may arise from prolonged exposure to loud sounds.

However, it is important to consider the potential drawbacks of using earplugs as well. One common concern is that earplugs may interfere with our ability to communicate effectively. While this can be true to some extent, modern earplugs are designed to provide noise reduction while still allowing for clear communication. For instance, there are specialized earplugs that filter out harmful noise frequencies while allowing speech and other important sounds to pass through.

Another factor to consider is the discomfort that some people may experience when wearing earplugs for extended periods. It is essential to find earplugs that fit properly and are comfortable to wear, as ill-fitting or uncomfortable earplugs may discourage regular use. Additionally, it's important to note that earplugs should not be worn excessively, as our ears also need some exposure to natural sounds for proper functioning.

In conclusion, earplugs can be a valuable tool in safeguarding your hearing in a noisy world. They offer numerous advantages, including noise reduction, portability, and availability. While there may be some drawbacks to using earplugs, such as potential communication barriers or discomfort, these can be mitigated by selecting the right type of earplugs and using them appropriately. Ultimately, by incorporating earplugs into your daily routine, you can preserve your auditory health and enjoy the sounds of life without worrying about long-term damage.

Earmuffs: Pros and Cons

As we navigate through the hustle and bustle of our daily lives, our ears are constantly bombarded with an array of sounds – some pleasant, while others can be detrimental to our hearing health. In this subchapter, we delve into the pros and cons of a popular hearing protection device – earmuffs. Whether you are a music enthusiast, a construction worker, or simply someone concerned about preserving your hearing, this discussion is relevant to everyone.

Let us first explore the advantages of earmuffs. One of the primary benefits is their ability to provide excellent noise reduction. Earmuffs are designed to cover the entire ear, creating a seal that blocks out external noise. This makes them highly effective in environments with high decibel levels, such as construction sites or airports. Furthermore, earmuffs offer a comfortable fit, as they do not exert direct pressure on the ear canal like earplugs do. This makes them ideal for individuals who may find earplugs uncomfortable or have difficulty inserting them correctly.

Another advantage of earmuffs is their versatility. Unlike earplugs, earmuffs can be quickly and easily shared among multiple individuals, making them a cost-effective option for workplaces or events where hearing protection is required. Additionally, earmuffs often come with adjustable bands, allowing for a personalized fit that ensures maximum comfort and protection.

However, like any other product, earmuffs also have their drawbacks. The first concern is their bulkiness. Due to their design, earmuffs can be cumbersome and may interfere with certain activities, such as wearing hats or helmets. This can be a significant inconvenience for individuals who require head protection in their line of work. Additionally, earmuffs may not be as discreet as earplugs, which can be tucked away in a pocket or purse when not in use.

Furthermore, while earmuffs excel at blocking out external noise, they can also limit one's ability to hear essential sounds, such as alarms or verbal communication. This can be a safety concern in certain situations, highlighting the importance of finding a balance between hearing protection and maintaining situational awareness.

In conclusion, earmuffs offer several advantages, such as excellent noise reduction, comfort, and versatility. However, their bulkiness and potential limitations to hearing certain sounds should also be considered. Ultimately, the choice between earmuffs and other hearing protection devices depends on individual preferences, the specific environment, and the level of hearing protection required. By understanding the pros and cons of earmuffs, individuals can make informed decisions to safeguard their hearing in our noisy world.

Custom-Made Ear Protection

In a world where noise pollution is becoming increasingly prevalent, protecting our hearing has never been more crucial. The delicate mechanisms of our ears are easily damaged by excessive noise, leading to irreversible hearing loss and other auditory problems. Thankfully, advancements in technology have paved the way for custom-made ear protection, offering a personalized solution to safeguard your hearing.

Custom-made ear protection, also known as customized earplugs or earmolds, provides a tailored fit to each individual's unique ear shape and size. Unlike generic earplugs, which often fail to provide a proper seal, custom-made options ensure maximum protection by effectively blocking out harmful noise while preserving the clarity of speech and other important sounds.

One of the primary advantages of custom-made ear protection is its ability to reduce noise to a safe level without compromising sound quality. Unlike foam or silicone earplugs, which can muffle sounds and create a sensation of being underwater, custom-made options allow for a more natural listening experience. This is especially beneficial for musicians, concert-goers, and individuals working in loud environments, as it enables them to enjoy the music or communicate effectively while minimizing the risk of hearing damage.

Additionally, custom-made ear protection offers enhanced comfort and extended wearability. The earmolds are made from soft, medical-grade materials that conform to the contours of the ear, ensuring a secure and comfortable fit. This eliminates the need for constant adjustments or readjustments, reducing the risk of discomfort or irritation, even during prolonged use.

Furthermore, custom-made ear protection can be designed to cater to specific needs and preferences. For instance, musicians can opt for filters that attenuate specific frequencies while maintaining balanced sound reproduction, allowing them to hear their music accurately and protect their hearing simultaneously. Similarly, individuals exposed to loud noises at work can choose earmolds that provide additional protection in specific frequency ranges, ensuring comprehensive coverage against harmful sound levels.

In conclusion, custom-made ear protection is an essential tool in safeguarding your hearing in a noisy world. Its personalized fit, superior sound quality, and enhanced comfort make it a valuable investment for individuals across all walks of life. Whether you are a musician, concert enthusiast, or simply someone concerned about preserving your hearing, custom-made ear protection serves as a reliable guardian for your precious ears. Take the proactive step today and embrace the power of custom-made ear protection to enjoy the world of sound while keeping your hearing intact.

Choosing the Right Hearing Protection for Different Situations

In our modern, noisy world, protecting our ears has never been more important. With constant exposure to loud sounds, whether it be from daily activities or specific environments, it is crucial to take the necessary steps to safeguard our hearing. But with so many options available, how do we choose the right hearing protection for different situations?

When it comes to selecting the appropriate hearing protection, one size does not fit all. Different situations call for different types of protection, tailored to the specific needs of our ears. Let's explore some common scenarios and the corresponding hearing protection options:

1. Occupational Noise: For individuals working in industries such as construction, manufacturing, or aviation, exposure to high levels of noise is a daily occurrence. In these situations, earmuffs or earplugs with high noise reduction ratings (NRR) are recommended. These provide a physical barrier to block out excessive noise and ensure maximum protection.

2. Concerts and Music Festivals: Music lovers often find themselves in settings with booming speakers and loud crowds. In such cases, musicians' earplugs or high-fidelity earplugs are ideal. These reduce noise levels without compromising the music's quality, allowing you to enjoy the experience while still protecting your ears.

3. Sporting Events: Whether you're attending a motorsport event or cheering for your favorite team in a stadium, the noise levels can be overwhelming. Here, custom-fit earplugs with acoustic filters are a great choice. These earplugs reduce the volume of sound while

maintaining clarity, so you can still hear the cheers and excitement without damaging your hearing.

4. DIY Projects at Home: Engaging in DIY projects often involves using power tools, which can generate significant noise levels. In this case, foam earplugs or earmuffs can provide adequate protection. They are easily accessible, affordable, and effectively reduce noise levels.

Remember, hearing protection is not just for professionals or those regularly exposed to loud noises. It is essential for everyone to take care of their ears, as even brief exposure to loud sounds can cause permanent damage. Investing in quality hearing protection is a small price to pay compared to the lifelong consequences of hearing loss.

When selecting hearing protection, it is crucial to consider comfort, fit, and effectiveness. Seek out products that are specifically designed for the intended situation, ensuring they meet safety standards and provide the desired level of noise reduction.

By choosing the right hearing protection for different situations, you can enjoy all aspects of life while preserving your precious sense of hearing. Don't wait until it's too late – start prioritizing your ear health today. Remember, prevention is always better than cure.

Chapter 6: Proper Usage and Maintenance of Hearing Protection

How to Wear Earplugs Correctly

In today's noisy world, protecting our hearing has become more important than ever. Whether you are a musician, a frequent concert-goer, or simply someone who wants to enjoy a good night's sleep, earplugs are an essential tool in safeguarding your ears. However, it is crucial to wear them correctly to ensure maximum effectiveness. This subchapter will guide you through the proper way of wearing earplugs, ensuring that you get the most out of this simple yet powerful hearing protection device.

1. Choose the Right Type of Earplug: With various types of earplugs available in the market, it is important to choose the one that suits your needs best. Foam earplugs are excellent for general use and provide a snug fit. Silicone earplugs are reusable and moldable, offering a customizable fit. For musicians or individuals who need to hear specific frequencies, musician's earplugs with interchangeable filters are an ideal choice.

2. Clean Your Hands: Before inserting earplugs, make sure your hands are clean to avoid any potential ear infections. Wash your hands thoroughly with soap and water or use hand sanitizer if washing facilities are not available.

3. Roll, Pull, and Seal: Start by rolling the earplug between your thumb and index finger to compress it. With your other hand, reach over your head and gently pull your ear upward and backward to straighten

the ear canal. Insert the compressed earplug into your ear canal and hold it in place for a few seconds while it expands and creates a seal.

4. Check for a Proper Seal: After inserting the earplugs, ensure they are properly sealed in your ears. Gently press on the outside of each earplug to confirm a snug fit. If you feel any air leakage or discomfort, remove them and try again.

5. Avoid Overinsertion: While a snug fit is crucial, avoid pushing the earplugs too far into your ear canal. Overinsertion may cause discomfort, pain, or even damage to the delicate structures of your ear.

6. Remove Correctly: When removing earplugs, remember to do so gently. Slowly and carefully pull the earplug out of your ear, ensuring not to jerk or twist it abruptly.

By following these steps, you can confidently wear earplugs correctly and provide your ears with the protection they deserve. Remember, proper usage of earplugs is essential for maintaining healthy hearing, reducing the risk of noise-induced hearing loss, and enjoying the sounds of life for years to come.

Putting on and Adjusting Earmuffs

Earmuffs are a fantastic tool for protecting your ears from the damaging effects of noise. Whether you work in a noisy environment, enjoy shooting sports, or simply want to safeguard your hearing in a bustling city, earmuffs can be your best friend. In this subchapter, we will guide you through the proper way of putting on and adjusting earmuffs to ensure maximum protection and comfort.

First and foremost, it is crucial to choose the right pair of earmuffs for your needs. When selecting earmuffs, consider the noise reduction rating (NRR) and ensure it meets the required standards for your intended use. Additionally, take into account the fit and comfort of the earmuffs. You want a pair that fits securely over your ears without causing discomfort or pressure points.

To put on earmuffs properly, start by holding the earmuff with both hands and ensure the headband is fully extended. Position the earmuffs over your head, allowing the cups to rest comfortably over your ears. The headband should fit snugly against the back of your head, ensuring a secure fit. Adjust the headband length if necessary to achieve a proper seal.

Once the earmuffs are in place, it's important to check for a good seal. A proper seal is crucial for effective noise reduction. Gently press the cups against your head to ensure they are creating a tight seal around your ears. You should feel a noticeable reduction in ambient noise once the seal is achieved.

Remember that earmuffs alone may not provide complete protection in extremely loud environments. If you are exposed to excessive noise levels, it is advisable to combine earmuffs with earplugs for added protection. This combination can provide a higher level of noise reduction, especially in hazardous environments.

It is important to adjust your earmuffs as needed throughout the day. Over time, the seal may loosen due to movement or sweat, compromising their effectiveness. Regularly check the fit of your earmuffs and readjust them as necessary to maintain a proper seal.

In conclusion, earmuffs are an essential tool for protecting your ears from excessive noise. By choosing the right pair, putting them on correctly, and ensuring a proper seal, you can effectively safeguard your hearing in a noisy world. Remember to adjust your earmuffs as needed to maintain their effectiveness throughout the day. Your ears deserve the utmost care and attention, and earmuffs are a valuable ally in preserving your hearing health.

Cleaning and Maintaining Hearing Protection Devices

Protecting our hearing is crucial in today's noisy world. Whether you work in a loud environment, enjoy attending concerts, or simply want to safeguard your ears, hearing protection devices play a vital role in maintaining healthy hearing. However, it is essential to clean and maintain these devices properly to ensure their effectiveness and longevity.

Cleaning your hearing protection devices is a simple yet important task that should be performed regularly. Depending on the type of device you use, there are various cleaning methods to consider. For disposable foam earplugs, you should discard them after each use and replace them with fresh ones. This prevents the buildup of dirt, earwax, and bacteria that can potentially lead to infections.

For reusable silicone earplugs or earmuffs, a gentle cleaning routine is necessary. Begin by wiping the exterior surfaces with a clean, damp cloth or mild soap. Avoid using harsh chemicals or abrasive materials that could damage the device. For removable silicone tips or cushions, these can usually be washed with warm water and mild soap. Ensure they are thoroughly dried before reattaching them to the device.

Additionally, it is crucial to regularly inspect your hearing protection devices for any signs of wear or damage. Check for cracks, tears, or deformities that may affect the device's ability to provide adequate protection. If you notice any issues, it is best to replace the device immediately to ensure continued effectiveness.

Proper storage is another key aspect of maintaining hearing protection devices. After cleaning and drying your devices, store them in a clean, dry container or case. This helps protect them from dust, moisture, and damage while also ensuring they remain hygienic for future use.

Remember to follow the manufacturer's instructions for cleaning and maintenance specific to your hearing protection device. These guidelines may differ depending on the type and brand of device you have chosen.

By diligently cleaning and maintaining your hearing protection devices, you can extend their lifespan and optimize their performance. Clean devices not only provide better protection for your ears but also contribute to a more comfortable and hygienic experience. Remember, healthy hearing begins with proper care of your hearing protection devices.

Ensuring a Proper Fit for Custom-Made Ear Protection

Custom-made ear protection is an essential tool in safeguarding your hearing in today's noisy world. Whether you are a musician, concert-goer, industrial worker, or simply someone who values their auditory health, investing in custom ear protection can make a significant difference in preserving your ears for years to come. However, it is crucial to understand that the effectiveness of these devices lies in their proper fit.

One of the most significant advantages of custom-made ear protection is that it is tailored specifically to your ears. Unlike generic earplugs or headphones, custom options are molded to fit the unique contours of your ear canal. This personalized fit ensures maximum comfort and noise reduction without compromising sound quality.

To ensure a proper fit for your custom-made ear protection, it is essential to work with a qualified audiologist or hearing professional. These experts have the knowledge and expertise to take precise measurements of your ears, ensuring that the earplugs or earmolds are accurately molded to your specifications.

During the fitting process, the audiologist will use specialized equipment to create an impression of your ear canal. This impression is then sent to a laboratory where the custom ear protection is manufactured. Once the earplugs or earmolds are ready, you will return for a final fitting to ensure they fit snugly and comfortably.

It is crucial to communicate any specific needs or concerns to the audiologist during the fitting process. Whether you require ear protection for a specific activity or have certain preferences, sharing this information will help the audiologist find the best solution for you. Remember, the more accurate the fit, the better the ear protection will perform.

Furthermore, it is essential to regularly check the fit of your custom-made ear protection. Over time, the shape of your ears may change due to factors such as weight loss, aging, or medical conditions. If you notice any discomfort or a decrease in noise reduction, it is recommended to consult with your audiologist for a refitting.

In conclusion, custom-made ear protection offers unparalleled comfort and effectiveness in preserving your hearing. By ensuring a proper fit through the assistance of a qualified audiologist, you can enjoy the benefits of personalized ear protection tailored to your unique needs. Invest in your auditory health today and embrace a quieter, safer world.

Chapter 7: Strategies for Hearing Conservation

Creating a Hearing Conservation Program

In today's noisy world, our ears are constantly bombarded with various sounds and noises. Whether it's the blaring horns of traffic, the loud music at concerts, or the constant use of headphones, our ears are under constant stress. It is crucial for everyone to understand the importance of protecting their hearing and take steps to prevent hearing loss. This subchapter aims to guide individuals in creating a Hearing Conservation Program, enabling them to safeguard their hearing and maintain healthy ears for years to come.

A Hearing Conservation Program involves a series of measures designed to prevent and reduce the risk of hearing loss. The program begins by raising awareness about the importance of hearing protection and educating individuals about the potential hazards of excessive noise exposure. This chapter provides readers with a comprehensive understanding of the risks associated with noise and the impact it can have on their ears.

The first step in creating a Hearing Conservation Program is to assess the noise levels in various environments. Whether it's at work, in recreational settings, or at home, identifying areas with excessive noise is crucial. By conducting noise assessments, individuals can determine the need for hearing protection devices, such as earplugs or earmuffs, in specific situations.

Once noise levels are assessed, the program emphasizes the importance of implementing engineering controls. These measures involve modifying the environment to reduce noise levels. For instance, using sound-absorbing materials or designing noise barriers can significantly decrease the impact of noise on one's ears.

Additionally, the chapter delves into the selection and proper use of hearing protection devices. It provides detailed information on different types of earmuffs and earplugs, highlighting their features, advantages, and limitations. The program encourages individuals to use appropriate hearing protection devices consistently, ensuring maximum effectiveness in noise reduction.

Regular hearing tests are an essential component of any Hearing Conservation Program. The subchapter emphasizes the significance of scheduling regular hearing screenings to monitor any changes in hearing ability. By detecting hearing loss early, individuals can take necessary steps to prevent further damage and seek appropriate treatment.

Lastly, the chapter emphasizes the need for ongoing education and training for individuals and organizations. By regularly updating knowledge about hearing conservation and providing training sessions on the proper use of hearing protection devices, the program ensures that everyone remains informed and equipped to protect their ears effectively.

In conclusion, the subchapter "Creating a Hearing Conservation Program" provides individuals of all backgrounds with a comprehensive guide to safeguarding their hearing. By understanding the risks associated with excessive noise exposure and implementing appropriate measures, everyone can take an active role in preserving their hearing health. With the implementation of a Hearing Conservation Program, individuals can enjoy a world of vibrant sounds without compromising their ear health.

Implementing Engineering Controls to Reduce Noise

In our modern world, noise has become an ever-present companion, with detrimental effects on our health and well-being. Excessive noise exposure can lead to hearing loss, stress, sleep disturbances, and even cardiovascular problems. While it may seem impossible to escape the clutches of noise, there are ways to mitigate its impact on our lives. One effective approach is to implement engineering controls to reduce noise, thereby safeguarding our precious hearing.

Engineering controls involve modifying the environment or equipment to reduce noise levels at the source, thus preventing its propagation and exposure to individuals. These measures can be applied in various settings, from industrial workplaces to our own homes. By understanding and implementing these controls, we can significantly decrease our exposure to harmful noise.

One of the fundamental engineering controls is the use of sound barriers and enclosures. These physical structures effectively block or absorb sound waves, preventing their transmission to the surrounding environment. In industrial settings, for example, installing enclosures around noisy machinery can contain the noise within a specific area, reducing its impact on workers. Similarly, sound barriers along highways can minimize the noise reaching nearby residential areas, providing much-needed tranquility.

Another effective strategy is the implementation of noise control materials. These materials are specifically designed to absorb or dampen sound energy, reducing its intensity. Acoustic panels, for instance, can be installed in offices, schools, or other public spaces to absorb sound reflections and create a quieter environment. Additionally, the use of noise-absorbing floor and ceiling materials can significantly minimize noise transmission between floors in buildings.

In some cases, engineering controls can involve modifying the design or operation of equipment. In the manufacturing industry, for example, engineers can design machines with noise reduction features, such as vibration isolation or soundproof enclosures. By reducing the noise emitted directly from the source, the need for personal protective equipment, like earplugs or earmuffs, can be minimized.

Implementing engineering controls to reduce noise is a vital step towards protecting our ears and overall well-being. Whether at work, home, or in public spaces, we have the power to create a quieter and healthier environment for ourselves and future generations. By understanding the principles of noise control and applying them effectively, we can safeguard our hearing in this noisy world we live in. Remember, it is never too late to take action and prioritize the health of our ears.

Administrative Controls for Hearing Protection

In our modern world, noise pollution has become an ever-present threat to our hearing health. From bustling cities to industrial workplaces, our ears are constantly bombarded with loud and potentially damaging sounds. However, there are measures that can be taken to safeguard our precious hearing. In this subchapter, we will explore the importance of administrative controls in hearing protection.

Administrative controls refer to the implementation of policies and procedures aimed at minimizing exposure to loud noise. These controls are crucial in various settings, including workplaces, schools, and even recreational areas. By establishing and enforcing administrative controls, we can mitigate the risk of noise-induced hearing loss.

One of the primary administrative controls is the implementation of noise control regulations. By setting limits on noise levels, organizations can ensure that their employees or visitors are not exposed to hazardous sound levels. This can involve identifying and addressing sources of excessive noise, such as machinery or equipment, through soundproofing or replacing them with quieter alternatives.

Another key aspect of administrative controls is the establishment of regular noise assessments. By conducting periodic measurements of noise levels, organizations can identify areas or activities that pose a potential risk to hearing health. Based on these assessments, appropriate measures can be taken to reduce noise exposure, such as modifying work schedules or providing hearing protection devices.

Training and education also play a vital role in administrative controls for hearing protection. By raising awareness about the dangers of noise exposure and providing guidance on how to effectively use hearing protection devices, individuals can take proactive steps in safeguarding their hearing. This education should be accessible to everyone, regardless of their occupation or age, as noise-induced hearing loss can affect individuals from all walks of life.

Furthermore, regular communication between employers, employees, and relevant stakeholders is essential. By fostering a culture of open dialogue, concerns related to noise exposure can be addressed promptly, and necessary adjustments can be made to further protect hearing health.

In conclusion, administrative controls are crucial in ensuring hearing protection in our noisy world. By implementing noise control regulations, conducting regular noise assessments, providing education and training, and fostering effective communication, we can safeguard our ears from the damaging effects of excessive noise. Remember, hearing health is essential for everyone, and by taking these administrative controls seriously, we can preserve our hearing for years to come.

Personal Protective Equipment (PPE) Policies and Procedures

As we navigate through the modern-day world, it is crucial to prioritize our health and safety. One area that often gets overlooked is the protection of our ears. In this subchapter, we will discuss the importance of Personal Protective Equipment (PPE) policies and procedures in safeguarding your hearing in a noisy world.

First and foremost, it is essential to understand the significance of PPE in preserving our hearing capabilities. PPE refers to any equipment or device worn to minimize exposure to hazardous noise levels. This can include earplugs, earmuffs, or noise-canceling headphones. By implementing PPE policies, we can effectively reduce the risk of noise-induced hearing loss and other auditory disorders.

The primary audience for this information is everyone. Whether you work in a loud industrial setting, attend concerts frequently, or simply enjoy listening to music with headphones, understanding and implementing PPE policies is vital for maintaining healthy ears.

One of the key aspects of PPE policies and procedures is education and awareness. By learning about the potential dangers of excessive noise and the benefits of using protective equipment, individuals can make informed decisions about their hearing health. This subchapter will provide comprehensive information on the different types of PPE available, their effectiveness, and how to use them correctly.

Additionally, we will delve into the importance of regular hearing screenings and the role they play in monitoring any changes or damage to our ears. By incorporating these screenings into your personal health routine, you can detect any hearing-related issues early on and take appropriate action.

Furthermore, this subchapter will outline best practices for implementing PPE policies in various environments. Whether you are an employer looking to protect your employees' hearing or an individual concerned about your own well-being, we will provide practical guidelines and procedures to ensure maximum effectiveness and compliance.

In conclusion, understanding and implementing PPE policies and procedures is essential for safeguarding your hearing in a noisy world. By taking the necessary steps to protect our ears, we can prevent long-term damage and maintain healthy hearing throughout our lives. This subchapter will serve as a comprehensive guide for individuals from all walks of life, offering practical advice and information to ensure the well-being of your ears. Remember, your hearing health is in your hands – protect it with PPE!

Chapter 8: The Role of Education and Awareness

Spreading Awareness about Hearing Conservation

In today's fast-paced and noisy world, our ears are constantly bombarded with excessive noise levels that can have a detrimental impact on our hearing health. It is crucial for everyone to understand the importance of hearing conservation and take proactive measures to safeguard their ears. This subchapter aims to spread awareness about the significance of preserving our hearing and provides practical tips on how to prevent hearing loss.

The human ear is an intricate organ that allows us to experience the beautiful symphony of sounds around us. However, prolonged exposure to loud noises can damage the delicate structures within the ear, leading to irreversible hearing loss. This can have a profound impact on our quality of life, affecting our ability to communicate, enjoy music, and even perform daily tasks. Therefore, taking steps to protect our ears is essential.

One of the key aspects of hearing conservation is understanding the concept of noise-induced hearing loss (NIHL). This type of hearing loss occurs when we are exposed to high decibel levels over an extended period. By educating ourselves and others about NIHL, we can make informed choices about our environment and take necessary precautions to prevent hearing damage.

To safeguard our ears, it is important to identify potentially harmful noise sources in our surroundings. These can include loud music concerts, construction sites, or even everyday activities like using power tools or listening to music through headphones at high volumes. By being mindful of these sources, we can limit our exposure to excessive noise and protect our hearing.

Utilizing hearing protection devices is another effective way to prevent hearing loss. Earplugs and earmuffs are readily available and can significantly reduce the impact of loud noises on our ears. Whether we are working in a noisy environment or attending a concert, wearing these protective gears can make a significant difference in preserving our hearing health.

Additionally, practicing safe listening habits is crucial for hearing conservation. Limiting the duration and volume of personal audio devices, taking breaks from noisy environments, and maintaining a healthy distance from loudspeakers are simple yet effective ways to protect our ears. By incorporating these habits into our daily lives, we can reduce the risk of developing hearing loss.

In conclusion, spreading awareness about hearing conservation is vital for everyone. By understanding the risks of noise-induced hearing loss and implementing preventive measures, we can safeguard our ears and preserve our hearing health. Remember, our ears are precious, and taking proactive steps to protect them is a lifelong investment in our well-being.

Educating Employees, Students, and the General Public

In today's noisy world, it is crucial to prioritize the health and wellbeing of our ears. The constant exposure to loud sounds, whether at work, school, or in public spaces, can lead to irreversible hearing damage. That is why it is essential to educate employees, students, and the general public about the importance of protecting their hearing.

One of the key aspects of educating individuals about hearing health is raising awareness about the potential risks associated with noise exposure. Many people are unaware that everyday activities, such as listening to loud music, using headphones at high volumes, or working in noisy environments, can have detrimental effects on their hearing. By highlighting these risks, we can empower individuals to take necessary precautions and make informed decisions to protect their ears.

For employees, it is crucial to provide comprehensive training and education programs in workplaces where noise levels are consistently high. By educating employees about the potential hazards of noise exposure and providing them with the knowledge and tools to protect their hearing, employers can create a safer and healthier work environment. This may include implementing noise control measures, such as soundproofing or regular maintenance of machinery, as well as promoting the use of personal protective equipment like earplugs or earmuffs.

In educational institutions, it is equally important to prioritize hearing health. Students, especially young children and teenagers, may not be aware of the potential risks associated with loud noises. Integrating hearing health education into the curriculum can help raise awareness and instill good hearing habits from an early age. This can include teaching students about safe listening practices, the importance of taking breaks from loud noises, and the potential long-term consequences of noise-induced hearing loss.

Beyond workplaces and schools, educating the general public about hearing health is crucial. Public awareness campaigns and initiatives can play a significant role in reaching a broader audience. By partnering with healthcare professionals, government organizations, and community leaders, we can disseminate information about hearing protection, safe listening practices, and available resources for those experiencing hearing loss.

In conclusion, educating employees, students, and the general public about the importance of protecting their hearing is paramount in today's noisy world. By raising awareness, providing training programs, and implementing public awareness campaigns, we can safeguard our ears and prevent irreversible hearing damage. Let us come together as a community to prioritize hearing health and create a quieter and safer world for everyone.

Promoting Hearing Health in the Community

In today's noisy world, it is crucial to prioritize and safeguard our hearing health. The ability to hear allows us to connect with others, experience the beauty of music, and navigate the world around us. However, with the increasing prevalence of loud environments and the use of personal audio devices, our ears are constantly exposed to potential harm. This subchapter aims to educate and empower individuals from all walks of life about the importance of preserving their hearing and promoting hearing health in their communities.

Understanding the anatomy and function of the ear is the first step towards hearing health awareness. The ear is a complex organ that consists of three main sections: the outer ear, middle ear, and inner ear. Each part plays a vital role in transmitting sound waves and converting them into electrical signals that our brain can interpret. By familiarizing ourselves with the ear's structure, we can better appreciate the importance of maintaining its health.

Noise-induced hearing loss (NIHL) is a prevalent and preventable condition that affects people of all ages. This section will delve into the various causes of NIHL, such as prolonged exposure to loud noises, recreational activities, and occupational hazards. It will also provide practical tips on how to protect our ears in these situations, such as using earplugs or earmuffs, taking breaks from noisy environments, and adjusting the volume of personal audio devices.

Beyond personal protection, promoting hearing health in the community involves raising awareness and advocating for change. This subchapter will explore the role of education campaigns, public policies, and community initiatives in fostering a culture of hearing health. It will highlight the importance of early detection and intervention through regular hearing screenings and encourage individuals to seek professional help if they notice any changes in their hearing ability.

Moreover, the chapter will emphasize the significance of inclusivity and accessibility in promoting hearing health. It will discuss how individuals with hearing impairments can be supported through assistive technologies, captioning services, and inclusive design practices. By creating a more inclusive environment, we can ensure that everyone, regardless of their hearing abilities, can fully participate in social, educational, and professional activities.

Ultimately, promoting hearing health in the community requires collective effort and individual responsibility. By empowering individuals with knowledge, providing practical tips for protection, and advocating for change, we can safeguard our hearing and create a healthier auditory environment for all. This subchapter aims to inspire and equip readers with the tools and information they need to become sound guardians of their own hearing and ambassadors of hearing health within their communities.

The Importance of Regular Hearing Check-ups

In our fast-paced and noisy world, it is all too easy to take our hearing for granted. We often fail to realize just how vital our ears are until we experience hearing loss or other hearing-related issues. That is why regular hearing check-ups are crucial for everyone, regardless of age or occupation. By prioritizing our auditory health, we can safeguard our hearing and ensure a better quality of life.

Our ears serve as the gateway to the sounds of the world around us. They enable us to communicate, enjoy music, and stay alert to potential dangers. However, prolonged exposure to loud noises, aging, and certain medical conditions can all contribute to hearing loss. Regular hearing check-ups can help identify any early signs of hearing loss and allow for timely intervention.

One of the primary benefits of regular hearing check-ups is the early detection of hearing problems. Like any health condition, the sooner hearing issues are identified, the better the chances of successful treatment. By detecting hearing loss in its early stages, healthcare professionals can develop personalized treatment plans, which may include hearing aids, cochlear implants, or other interventions. These interventions can significantly improve the quality of life for individuals experiencing hearing loss.

Regular hearing check-ups also play a crucial role in preventing further damage to our hearing. By monitoring our auditory health over time, healthcare professionals can identify any alarming trends or changes in our hearing ability. They can then provide guidance on how to protect our ears from excessive noise, whether through the use of earplugs or adopting healthy listening habits.

Moreover, regular hearing check-ups are essential for maintaining overall well-being. Untreated hearing loss has been linked to decreased cognitive function, social isolation, and even mental health issues. By staying on top of our auditory health, we can reduce the risk of these negative consequences and enjoy a more fulfilling and connected life.

In conclusion, given the vital role our ears play in our daily lives, regular hearing check-ups are of utmost importance for everyone. By prioritizing our auditory health, we can detect hearing problems early, receive timely treatment, and prevent further damage. Don't wait until your hearing is compromised – schedule your next hearing check-up and start taking proactive steps to safeguard your hearing today. Remember, healthy ears lead to a healthier and happier life.

Chapter 9: The Future of Ear Protection

Advancements in Hearing Protection Technology

In our modern world, it is becoming increasingly important to safeguard our hearing from the harmful effects of noise pollution. Whether it's the constant blaring of traffic, the cacophony of construction sites, or the thunderous roar of music concerts, our ears are constantly exposed to high decibel levels that can lead to irreversible damage. Fortunately, advancements in hearing protection technology have enabled us to take control of our auditory well-being like never before.

One of the most significant advancements in hearing protection technology is the development of noise-canceling headphones. These innovative devices use microphones to pick up external sounds and then generate a counter sound wave that cancels out the incoming noise. This allows users to enjoy their favorite music or podcasts at lower volumes, reducing the risk of hearing damage. Noise-canceling headphones are particularly beneficial for frequent travelers or individuals working in noisy environments.

Another exciting advancement is the advent of custom-fit earplugs. Unlike generic foam earplugs that provide a one-size-fits-all solution, custom-fit earplugs are tailor-made to fit the unique contours of an individual's ear. This ensures a snug fit and maximum comfort, while also providing superior noise reduction. Custom-fit earplugs are ideal for musicians, industrial workers, and anyone who wants to protect their hearing without sacrificing sound quality or communication abilities.

For those who enjoy live music or attend loud events, musician's earplugs offer a perfect solution. These earplugs are specially designed to attenuate harmful noise levels while preserving the integrity of sound. Musicians and concert-goers can now enjoy the full experience of live performances without compromising their hearing health.

Advancements in hearing protection technology have also extended to the realm of smartphone applications. There are now apps available that measure ambient noise levels in real-time and provide users with personalized recommendations for hearing protection. These apps can also track an individual's noise exposure over time, empowering users to make informed decisions about their auditory health.

In conclusion, the advancements in hearing protection technology have revolutionized the way we safeguard our ears in a noisy world. Whether it's noise-canceling headphones, custom-fit earplugs, musician's earplugs, or smartphone apps, there is a solution for everyone. By taking advantage of these advancements, we can protect our hearing and ensure a healthier auditory future.

Potential Innovations in Noise Reduction

In today's fast-paced world, noise pollution has become an unavoidable part of our daily lives. From bustling city streets to crowded public transportation, our ears are constantly bombarded with excessive noise levels that can have detrimental effects on our hearing. However, there is hope on the horizon as technological advancements continue to pave the way for potential innovations in noise reduction. In this subchapter, we will explore some of these groundbreaking innovations that hold the promise of safeguarding your hearing in a noisy world.

One of the most exciting innovations in noise reduction is the development of intelligent noise-cancelling headphones. These headphones utilize advanced algorithms and built-in microphones to detect ambient noise and generate an equal and opposite sound wave, effectively canceling out the external noise. This technology allows you to enjoy your favorite music or podcasts without having to crank up the volume to dangerous levels, protecting your ears from potential damage.

Another promising innovation is the use of active noise control in vehicles. Car manufacturers are now incorporating noise-canceling systems into their vehicles, which actively monitor and counteract engine, wind, and road noise. By reducing the overall noise levels within the cabin, these systems aim to provide a more peaceful and comfortable driving experience while preventing long-term hearing damage.

In the architectural world, innovative building materials are being developed to reduce noise pollution. Advanced sound-absorbing materials can be used in the construction of buildings, minimizing the transmission of noise between rooms and from the outside environment. This not only creates a quieter indoor space but also reduces the need for excessive use of personal hearing protection.

Furthermore, advancements in hearing aid technology are revolutionizing the way we address hearing loss caused by noise exposure. Smart hearing aids now come equipped with sophisticated noise reduction algorithms that can differentiate between speech and background noise, amplifying the former while suppressing the latter. This ensures that individuals with hearing impairments can effectively communicate in noisy environments, improving their overall quality of life.

As technology continues to evolve, the potential for further innovations in noise reduction is vast. From wearable devices to noise-mapping applications, the future holds exciting possibilities for protecting our ears in a noisy world. However, it is essential to remember that while these innovations can play a significant role in minimizing noise pollution, personal awareness and responsible behavior are equally crucial in safeguarding our hearing. By embracing these innovations and adopting healthy hearing habits, we can strive towards a quieter and safer world for everyone.

In conclusion, potential innovations in noise reduction offer hope for a future where our ears are protected from the damaging effects of noise pollution. From intelligent noise-cancelling headphones to advanced building materials, these innovations aim to create quieter environments and enhance our overall auditory well-being. By staying informed and embracing these advancements, we can take proactive steps to safeguard our hearing in a noisy world.

Research and Development in Hearing Conservation

In today's noisy world, our ears face an increasing threat of damage and hearing loss. However, thanks to continuous research and development in the field of hearing conservation, we now have a better understanding of how to safeguard our hearing and prevent further damage. This subchapter delves into the various advancements in research and development that have revolutionized the way we protect our ears.

One of the most significant breakthroughs in hearing conservation research is the development of advanced hearing protection devices. These devices are designed to reduce the intensity of loud sounds without compromising our ability to hear important sounds such as speech or music. With the help of cutting-edge technology, researchers have created earplugs and earmuffs that offer superior noise reduction capabilities while still allowing for clear communication.

Additionally, the study of noise-induced hearing loss has led to the discovery of new preventive measures. Researchers have found that certain vitamins and minerals, such as antioxidants, can mitigate the harmful effects of noise exposure on our ears. These findings have paved the way for the development of specialized supplements and dietary recommendations that can support hearing health and reduce the risk of hearing loss.

Furthermore, research has also shed light on the importance of early detection and intervention in hearing loss. Improved diagnostic tools and techniques have enabled healthcare professionals to identify hearing problems at an early stage, allowing for timely interventions and treatment. This has significantly contributed to preserving and enhancing the quality of life for individuals with hearing impairments.

In recent years, the field of hearing conservation has witnessed advancements in the area of assistive listening devices. These devices, such as hearing aids and cochlear implants, have undergone significant improvements in terms of functionality and comfort. They now offer enhanced sound quality and customization options, catering to the specific needs of individuals with hearing loss.

Moreover, ongoing research is exploring innovative therapies and regenerative treatments that have the potential to restore hearing in individuals with severe hearing loss or deafness. Stem cell research, gene therapy, and cochlear implant advancements are some of the exciting areas that hold promise for the future of hearing restoration.

In conclusion, the continuous research and development efforts in the field of hearing conservation have brought about significant advancements in protecting our ears from noise-induced damage. From advanced hearing protection devices and preventive measures to improved diagnostics and assistive listening devices, the field has made great strides in preserving and restoring hearing. As we move forward, it is crucial to stay informed about these developments and prioritize our hearing health in order to enjoy a noise-free and fulfilling life.

Promising Strategies for Future Ear Protection

In our modern, bustling world, our ears are constantly bombarded with various sources of noise. From bustling city streets to blaring headphones, our ears are under constant assault. As a result, it is becoming increasingly important to safeguard our hearing and protect our ears from potential damage.

Fortunately, advancements in technology and innovative strategies offer promising solutions for future ear protection. These strategies aim to provide effective and convenient ways to preserve our hearing in the face of everyday noise pollution.

One such strategy is the development of advanced noise-canceling technologies. These technologies utilize microphones and algorithms to actively reduce unwanted ambient noise, allowing us to enjoy our favorite music or engage in conversations without having to increase the volume to dangerous levels. Noise-canceling headphones and earbuds are already widely available, and with further advancements, they will become even more effective and accessible to everyone.

Another promising strategy lies in the development of custom-fit ear protection. Traditionally, earplugs and earmuffs have been the primary means of protecting our ears in loud environments. However, these generic solutions often provide an imperfect fit, compromising their effectiveness. Custom-fit ear protection, on the other hand, can be tailored to fit each individual's unique ear shape, ensuring optimal comfort and noise reduction. With advancements in 3D printing and personalized manufacturing, we can expect to see more affordable and accessible custom-fit ear protection options in the future.

Furthermore, education and awareness play a crucial role in preventing hearing damage. By promoting the importance of ear protection and providing information on the potential risks of noise exposure, we can empower individuals to take proactive measures to safeguard their hearing. This includes encouraging the use of ear protection in loud environments, such as concerts and construction sites, and educating individuals about the potential long-term consequences of untreated hearing loss.

In conclusion, the future of ear protection holds great promise. With the development of advanced noise-canceling technologies, custom-fit ear protection, and increased awareness, we can safeguard our hearing in an increasingly noisy world. By adopting these strategies, we can ensure that our ears remain healthy and functional, allowing us to fully enjoy the sounds of life for years to come. Remember, protecting your ears today means preserving your hearing for a lifetime.

Chapter 10: Conclusion and Resources

Recap of Key Points

Throughout "The Sound Guardian: Safeguarding Your Hearing in a Noisy World," we have explored the importance of protecting our ears and preventing hearing loss in today's noisy environment. In this final subchapter, let's recap the key points that every one, regardless of age or occupation, should keep in mind to maintain healthy ears.

First and foremost, understanding the detrimental effects of loud noise on our hearing is crucial. We have learned that prolonged exposure to loud sounds, such as music concerts, construction sites, or even the constant use of headphones, can lead to irreversible damage to our ears. This damage can manifest as hearing loss, tinnitus (ringing in the ears), or hyperacusis (increased sensitivity to sound). Therefore, it is essential to be mindful of our daily noise exposure and take steps to protect our ears from excessive noise.

One of the most effective ways to safeguard our hearing is through the use of ear protection devices. We have discussed the various options available, such as earplugs and earmuffs, that can significantly reduce noise levels and prevent hearing damage. Remember, it is not just industrial workers or musicians who need to protect their ears – everyone, from children to adults, should consider using ear protection in noisy environments.

Additionally, we have emphasized the importance of maintaining good ear hygiene. Regular cleaning of our ears is essential, but it is crucial to do it safely. Inserting objects like cotton swabs or sharp instruments into the ear canal can damage delicate structures and even push wax deeper, leading to complications. Instead, gentle cleaning with a washcloth or seeking professional help when necessary is recommended.

Furthermore, we have explored the role of diet and lifestyle in promoting healthy ears. Consuming a balanced diet rich in nutrients like omega-3 fatty acids, antioxidants, and vitamins can support overall ear health. Regular exercise, stress management, and avoiding smoking and excessive alcohol consumption also contribute to maintaining good hearing.

Finally, we encourage every one to prioritize regular hearing screenings. Early detection of any hearing problems can prevent further damage and facilitate timely intervention. Visiting an audiologist or healthcare professional for periodic check-ups is essential, especially for those at higher risk, such as individuals with a family history of hearing loss or those exposed to hazardous noise regularly.

In conclusion, "The Sound Guardian" has provided a comprehensive guide on how to safeguard your hearing in a noisy world. By understanding the dangers of excessive noise, using ear protection, practicing proper ear hygiene, adopting a healthy lifestyle, and getting regular screenings, we can all take proactive steps towards preserving our precious sense of hearing. Remember, healthy ears lead to a better quality of life for every one!

Additional Resources for Hearing Conservation

In our modern world, where noise pollution is on the rise, it is crucial to prioritize the health of our ears and safeguard our hearing. While the previous chapters of this book have provided you with valuable information and strategies to protect your ears, it is important to be aware of the additional resources available to aid in your hearing conservation journey. Whether you are an individual concerned about your own hearing or a professional working in the field of audiology, these resources can provide you with further guidance and support.

1. Audiologists and Hearing Healthcare Professionals: Audiologists are highly trained professionals who specialize in the prevention, diagnosis, and treatment of hearing disorders. If you have concerns about your hearing, seeking the help of an audiologist or hearing healthcare professional is recommended. These experts can conduct comprehensive hearing evaluations, provide personalized advice, and recommend appropriate hearing protection devices.

2. Hearing Conservation Programs: Many organizations and workplaces have implemented hearing conservation programs to protect the hearing of their employees. These programs typically include regular hearing screenings, noise level assessments, and education on hearing protection. If you are an employer or part of a safety committee, consider implementing such a program to ensure the well-being of your employees' ears.

3. Hearing Protection Devices: There is a wide range of hearing protection devices available in the market, including earplugs and earmuffs. These devices can help reduce the impact of loud noises on

your hearing. It is essential to choose the right hearing protection device based on your specific needs and the noise levels you are exposed to regularly. Consult an audiologist or hearing healthcare professional to find the best option for you.

4. Online Resources: The internet provides a wealth of information on hearing conservation. Numerous websites and online forums provide valuable resources, articles, and research studies related to hearing health. You can find information on the latest advancements in hearing protection technology, tips for preventing hearing loss, and stories of individuals who have successfully protected their hearing.

Remember, hearing conservation is a lifelong commitment, and it is never too early or too late to start prioritizing the health of your ears. By utilizing the additional resources mentioned above, you can enhance your understanding of hearing conservation and take proactive steps to protect your ears in our noisy world.

Taking Action: Steps Towards Protecting Your Hearing

In today's noisy world, our ears constantly face the risk of damage and hearing loss. Fortunately, there are several steps you can take to protect your hearing and ensure a lifetime of healthy hearing. By being proactive and implementing these measures, you can safeguard your ears from the detrimental effects of excessive noise exposure.

The first and most crucial step towards protecting your hearing is to become aware of the potential risks that surround you. Identify the sources of loud noise in your daily life, such as construction sites, concerts, or even your personal listening devices. Understanding the decibel levels and duration of exposure to these sounds will allow you to take appropriate action.

One of the simplest yet effective ways to protect your hearing is by using earplugs or earmuffs. These devices act as a barrier against excessive noise, reducing the intensity of sound reaching your ears. Whether you are attending a concert, operating machinery, or even mowing the lawn, wearing ear protection can significantly minimize the risk of hearing damage.

Additionally, it is crucial to practice safe listening habits when using personal audio devices. Limit the volume to a level that allows you to hear background sounds and conversations without straining. Taking breaks from continuous use and using noise-cancelling headphones can also help reduce the risk of hearing loss.

Regular hearing check-ups are essential for maintaining ear health. Schedule appointments with an audiologist or healthcare professional to monitor your hearing abilities and detect any potential issues early on. Early intervention can make a significant difference in preventing further damage and maximizing treatment options.

Moreover, adopting a healthy lifestyle can indirectly contribute to protecting your hearing. Exercise regularly, maintain a balanced diet, and manage stress levels. These habits promote overall well-being, including the health of your ears.

Lastly, educating others about the importance of hearing protection is crucial. Spread awareness among your friends, family, and colleagues. Encourage them to take action and prioritize their hearing health.

By taking these steps towards protecting your hearing, you are actively safeguarding one of your most precious senses. Remember, prevention is always better than cure. Start implementing these measures today and create a soundscape that preserves your hearing for years to come.

Final Thoughts and Encouragement for Safeguarding Your Hearing

Protecting our hearing is of utmost importance in today's noisy world. Our ears are invaluable sensory organs that allow us to experience the beauty of sound and connect with the world around us. However, they are also delicate and vulnerable to damage caused by excessive noise exposure. As we conclude this book, "The Sound Guardian: Safeguarding Your Hearing in a Noisy World," let us reflect on the importance of hearing preservation and find encouragement to embark on this crucial journey.

First and foremost, it is essential to acknowledge that everyone, regardless of age or occupation, needs to prioritize their hearing health. Whether you are a musician, a construction worker, a student, or simply someone who enjoys listening to music, understanding the risks associated with noise exposure is vital. By taking proactive steps to safeguard our hearing, we can prevent irreversible damage and maintain our quality of life.

One of the key takeaways from this book is the significance of education and awareness. We must educate ourselves and others about the impact of noise on our hearing. By understanding the decibel levels that can cause harm and learning to recognize hazardous situations, we can make informed choices to protect our ears. Additionally, spreading this knowledge among friends, family, and coworkers can help create a culture of hearing health and encourage collective action.

Implementing practical strategies in our daily lives is another crucial aspect of hearing protection. Using earplugs or earmuffs in noisy environments, turning down the volume on our personal electronic devices, and taking regular breaks from loud activities are simple yet effective ways to reduce our exposure to harmful noise. It is important to remember that prevention is always better than cure when it comes to hearing loss.

Finally, let us remember that safeguarding our hearing is an ongoing process. It requires commitment, perseverance, and a willingness to make necessary lifestyle changes. Regular hearing check-ups with a qualified audiologist are essential to monitor our hearing health and detect any early signs of damage. By prioritizing our hearing, we are investing in a future of better communication, improved mental well-being, and enhanced overall quality of life.

In conclusion, as we bid farewell, I encourage each and every one of you to be the guardian of your own hearing. Take the knowledge and insights gained from this book and apply them in your life. Remember, our ears are irreplaceable, and their protection should be our utmost priority. Together, let us create a world where the beauty of sound can be enjoyed by all, for generations to come.

www.ingramcontent.com/pod-product-compliance
Lightning Source LLC
LaVergne TN
LVHW051957060526
838201LV00059B/3703